## Belly Button Bliss

A Small Collection of Happy Birth Stories

# Belly Button Bliss

A Small Collection of Happy Birth Stories

Edited by
## Jennifer Derryberry Mann

FAIRVIEW PRESS
Minneapolis

Published by Fairview Press, 2450 Riverside Avenue, Minneapolis, Minnesota 55454. Fairview Press is a division of Fairview Health Services, a community-focused health system, affiliated with the University of Minnesota, providing a complete range of services, from the prevention of illness and injury to care for the most complex medical conditions. For a free current catalog of Fairview Press titles, please call toll-free 1-800-544-8207. Or visit our Web site at www.fairviewpress.org.

**Library of Congress Cataloging-in-Publication Data**
Belly button bliss : a small collection of happy birth stories / Compiled and edited by Jennifer Derryberry Mann.

  p. cm.
 ISBN 978-1-57749-230-6 (alk. paper)
 1. Childbirth—Popular works. 2. Childbirth—Anecdotes. I. Mann, Jennifer Derryberry.
 RG525.B447 2010
 618.2—dc22

                    2010005783

Printed in the United States of America
First Printing: August 2010
14  13  12  11  10      7  6  5  4  3  2  1

Design by Ginkgo Creative, Inc. (ginkgocreative.com)

for mamas and babies everywhere

and for the brightest lights in my life

*Anabel and Alia*

and the one who holds us on an even keel

through pregnancy, birth, and beyond

trusted husband, friend, and father

*Scotty*

# Contents

## Hospital Births

# Home Births

# Extra Special Births

TWINS, CESAREAN SECTION,
VAGINAL BIRTH AFTER CESAREAN, ADOPTION

# Why Birth Stories Matter

**Mamas-to-be get a lot of things** while pregnant: advice, some good, some bad. Heartburn, all bad. Gifts, some cute, some not. All well intended. And then there are the birth stories that women share with each other. Like the gifts, they're meant to be helpful. But not all of them are as uplifting as a pretty pastel-wrapped package.

While I was pregnant with my first baby, a couple of acquaintances recounted their scary moments in labor. Surely, they meant well. Perhaps they thought knowing what to watch out for might help me. It's not that I had blinders on, or unrealistic expectations about birth. Indeed, like many expectant mothers, I was aware of the range of experiences and outcomes—good and not so good— possible in labor and birth. I had read up on the risks and sat through all the childbirth classes and talked with my care providers seemingly ad nauseam. But when it came to talking about birth with family, friends, acquaintances, and even strangers, I had but one wish: inspiration and encouragement, please!

It turns out that many pregnant women feel that way, and some of them have shared their happy birth stories in this book. They all did so for one main reason, which mama Maureen Hunt sums up nicely: "We need more good birth stories out there!"

Every birth is, at its core, essentially, wondrously, the same. This efficient little haiku, jotted down by my friend Erika Rasmusson Janes, captures the gist perfectly:

*water breaks, pain comes*
*push, push, push, push, push, push, push*
*then baby, and love*

And yet every birth story is unique. Some of us labor quickly, others more slowly. We handle pain differently, but we all feel the intensity. We relish the moment our babies enter the world, sometimes with great relief, other times with great jubilation. We see elements of ourselves in each other's stories while marveling at the differences in our experiences.

As for the birth stories of my two girls, my first, Anabel, was born quickly on the morning of her due date, October 8. She weighed 8 pounds 3 ounces, and measured 20 inches. Her birth was a powerful event, very focused, and full of intensity. Alia was born one week after her due date, on the afternoon of August 6. She weighed 9 pounds 15.8 ounces, and measured 21 inches. I spent a sweet morning laboring with her, enjoying the heat pack on my low back and the aromatherapy my doula provided. When it came time to move through the final phase of labor that afternoon, birth was every bit as powerful, focused, and intense as I remembered from two years before.

I had natural childbirths with both girls, at a hospital with the help of a midwife. That was a good arrangement for my husband and me, offering peace of mind for our families and reduced risk of medical intervention for me and my girls. With both births, I was dilated to about 7 or 8 centimeters when I arrived at the hospital, and each time, delivered about ninety minutes after making the slow, waddling walk from the emergency entrance to the maternity floor.

Birth happens fast and a little hard at my house, so I do remember the pain! But it doesn't define my girls' births, or my memory of those two amazing days. Of course the car rides to the hospital were ridiculous. The "ring of fire" is everything it sounds like it could be. And that moment before baby arrives feels like, well, what it feels like when two beings attempt to occupy the same space at the same time. Crushing, compacted, what-oh-what-have-I-gotten-myself-into? There was one contraction, in particular, with Alia that I will never forget! Surely it lasted twenty minutes!

This is what I remember most, and hold dear, about birth: The experience was incredibly satisfying, as though I had expressed my deepest truth, and the world was delighted by that, *by me*, by these perfect babies.

Ultimately, I created this book because I believe passionately in women's intuitive wisdom about birth, the depths of our hearts, the strength of our bodies. I believe birth is most satisfying when women are informed and intentional about it—whether the choice is made for an epidural or no drugs at all, a home birth or a hospital birth, an OB or a midwife. It's important that women are at peace with their birth experiences, because birth is a transformative moment in a woman's life, whether she's conscious of that or not.

Birth changes you. And when you have ample support, lots of encouragement, and a positive frame of mind, the transformation is more likely to be a satisfying one.

Birth is top of mind for me, in part because I teach prenatal yoga. I love watching moms-to-be move through their pregnancy, gaining confidence in themselves, delighting in their bodies, wondering about the life growing inside them, both eager and a little anxious to meet this new person. In class, I ask moms to hold "Goddess pose"—a high, wide-legged squat—for several minutes near the end of each practice. It's not easy, and neither is birth, I tell them. It's intense. You shake. You sweat. You may think you can't do it, but here you are: beautiful and breathing, taking your just-right place in the long line of women who have birthed before you, holding a space for the mamas in the world who are birthing right now, and leading the way for the women who will birth after you. Women know—our bodies, our babies, our hearts know—how to birth; sometimes we just need a sweet reminder about what is possible.

The stories collected here are meant to be that sweet reminder. As I talked with the women who contributed to this anthology, I was fascinated by how widely they differ in their experience of the physical and emotional effort of birth. What stayed with me as I read each story is what I hope will stay with you, too: No matter the details of your birth, from the seemingly relentless pressure of a contraction to the elation of feeling your baby emerge into the world, from the pain pain pain to the belly button bliss—especially because of that moment of bliss—joy awaits.

# Hospital Births

Mama
Courtney Gordon Hay

**Baby**
Andra June
born October 29 at 5:23 a.m.
7 pounds 3 ounces
19 inches

# You Can Do Anything for a Day!

**I labored for twenty-eight hours** to bring Andra June into this world, and I learned that you can do anything for a day! This is just one of the many things I've learned from labor, birth, and motherhood.

I learned...

- *that my body knew exactly what to do and, even more important, to trust in birth as a natural process.*
- *how to focus all my energy on the image of my opening cervix.*
- *how to tap into my inner warrior.*
- *how helpful rocking on a birth ball can be through transition.*

Through my husband's tears, I learned that birth can have as great of an emotional effect on a father as it does on a mother.

I learned...

- *that you can fall asleep between pushes and that the final one is followed by the greatest sense of triumph.*
- *that after birth your belly feels like marshmallow cream.*
- *that no feeling compares to your newborn lying on your belly, looking into your eyes, or grasping your finger for the first time.*
- *that giving birth is the most miraculous experience in the world.*

Because of my beautiful, healthy baby girl, I gained a deep appreciation for every mother, no matter how her child came into this world. I gained a love so deep and intense I could never have imagined my heart big enough to contain it. I now know I can do anything. I brought a child into the world, and I am a mother.

Mama
Kirsten Ellenbogen

**Baby**
Ezra
born October 29 at 1:35 a.m.
8 pounds 10 ounces
21½ inches

# A Singular, Clear Feeling

**No one tells you that** your body keeps producing amniotic fluid, so when my water broke with my second baby, I sat around much of the day as I had with my first: trying not to leak too much.

After twelve hours of minor, irregular labor pains, my midwife asked me to come to the hospital. I was given a gentle once-over and sent home. We all agreed my contractions weren't that impressive. They did promise to hold a bed for me, wanting me back at the hospital within twenty-four hours of my water breaking.

A couple of hours later, the contractions became stronger and more regular. Between breathing, backrubs, and my birthing ball I did well for the next hour. When the pain-reducing techniques weren't working so well anymore, we called our doula for help. She asked me to describe the pain in more detail; a contraction started, so I handed the phone to my husband, Charles. I must have sounded intense, because our doula suggested we meet at the hospital.

We had been told numerous times that we would really know when labor was progressing because I'd feel miserable even between contractions. But we still felt rather relaxed. Charles had me laughing and smiling. The drive to the hospital was short (but bumpy!); we parked in the garage and made the long walk through the tunnel to the maternity ward.

This took forever. Five steps, and a pause for contractions. Another five steps, and more contractions. It wasn't like the movies; at 1 a.m., no one comes running with a wheelchair.

We stopped at the maternity check-in desk, but the next contraction actually made me yip. We were sent directly to the birthing room. I chatted with the nurse briefly and tried to give the urine sample she'd asked for, but I was overcome by a need to push. That was the clearest, most singular feeling I have ever had.

I gripped the wall. "I need to push!" I yelled. Charles ran into the hall, and whatever he said brought a lot of people running! With some convincing, I let go of the wall and made my way onto the bed. Pushing went quickly, and about five minutes later, our son Ezra was born, pink and loud. I've never felt so confident and sure of myself as I did in those few minutes.

**Mama**
Tricia Spitzmueller

**Baby**
Mary Christina
born March 20 at 6:47 p.m.
8 pounds 11 ounces
21 inches

# I Love You, Just Because

**I have five children, and** my last birth was definitely the most fun.

Field trip on bumpy school bus to Minnesota State Capitol and Governor's Mansion with my preschooler—who was supposedly my last of four!

Too many bumps and 500 steps up the Capitol building. Sat down on a chair in the mansion with sudden contractions, expecting my water to break. Baby's not due for a week. What's up?

More of the bumpy bus home.

My best friend—a nurse—and her son were part of the trip. She sees me wince. Promises to "be right back" to take me to the hospital after she drops her son off. I try to call my husband. This is harder than it sounds: no cell phones in 1986, and he's traveling for business. He's not at his last account, nor his next account, which is a hundred miles away.

Friend returns to take me to the hospital. My twelve-year-old babysits his siblings, who are just coming home from school.

Off I go!

My friend drops me off at the hospital, then returns to my house to bring my other four children to the hospital. They'd all taken the birthing classes and wanted to be there.

Contractions are coming very quickly.

Miraculously, thankfully, my husband feels a sudden nudge to "go home" even as he is driving to his next account. He calls home. "Mom's in the hospital!!!!" the kids excitedly scream.

Panic! Husband drives (like a maniac!) immediately to the hospital. He arrives five minutes before the birth, catches the baby, cuts the cord, and greets our other four children as they walk into the birth room.

My oldest son asks, "Can I hold her?" And with his littlest sister in his arms, he starts to tear up.

"Why are you crying, Matt?"

"Because I love her so much."

A teachable moment! "Why do you love her? Is it because she will grow up to be so smart, or to be a scientist, or a famous dancer?"

"*Mom*," he says. "I don't know what she will be, I just know that I love her!"

"Yes, Matt," I say. "That is how I love you too, and each of your siblings. I love you *just because*. Love isn't something you earn. It just is."

Mama
Julie Moon

**Baby**
Scarlett
born February 28 at 11:11 a.m.
8 pounds 13 ounces
21¾ inches

# A Whole New Person Is in the World!

I awake around 3:45 a.m. on my due date with contractions about six minutes apart. A terrible storm rages outside. I call my mother and my best friend, Stephanie, to give them time enough to arrive for Scarlett's birth.

My husband, Joe, is awake too, fixing a snack. My son, Jackson, is cozy and safe at his grandparents' house, where he'd gone to spend the night when I recognized the signs of early labor the afternoon before. Mom and Stephanie arrive by 5 a.m.

"I think Scarlett is going to be born today," I whisper to my daughter Savannah when I go in to wake her. She pops her head right up, so excited! Soon after, my photographer friend, Tracey, arrives.

We laugh a lot, focusing on fun rather than the contractions. By 6:15 a.m., I'm contracting every three minutes or so. We call the midwife to alert her, and thirty minutes later, we're on our way to the hospital. Scarlett, it seems, will be arriving on her due date, something that only 4 percent of babies do! By 7 a.m., we're at the hospital.

Now the rain outside is calm and peaceful. I'm more than 5 centimeters dilated, and Scarlett is head down and waiting. Savannah sits with Stephanie, playing games and reading books. Tracey waits and watches, at ease in a rocking chair in the corner. Mom and I answer questions for the nurse, and Joe waits patiently for me to need his support.

When I birth, my thighs burn during contractions, and I need a catnap. Soon, it's time for both. Joe rubs the top of my thighs, melting the pain and seemingly shortening my contractions. I lean over the bed and moan through each rubdown, then stand back up and chat and laugh, sharing stories of birthing Jackson and Savannah, and enjoying the company of the wonderful people experiencing this birth with me. Then it's time for that catnap.

Tired, I climb into bed and doze for about twenty minutes. When I awake, everyone agrees things are picking up. By 9:45 a.m., I sound "transitional" in my moans. After one contraction, Savannah passes me a note that says, "Mommy, that one was loud!"

It's 10:06 a.m., and my pants are off, a sure sign that birth is near! I never labor in a gown, always in comfortable yoga pants and a shirt. When things heat up, the pants come off. I began talking to my intact bag of waters: "Release, please release," knowing this would speed things along. At 10:58 a.m., I ask Susan, my midwife, to break my water. Scarlett's head is so far down that nothing much seems to happen.

Following Susan's advice, my mom steps in to help. She places her gloved hand over my perineum and offers firm support as I push on my hands and knees. Soon, Scarlett's head fills her hand, and at 11:11 a.m., my girl arrives! One hand is up by her head waving, and she cries so strongly. Once Scarlett's head and shoulders are out and the cord untangled from her, Mom lifts her up a bit so I can pull her the rest of the way out.

Big sister Savannah says it best: "A whole new person is in the world!"

Indeed! Scarlett weighs an impressive 8 pounds 13 ounces—my biggest baby by more than a pound!

She's beautiful, plump, and ruddy, with medium brown hair. Savannah says, "I can't believe I'm going to do that someday." And I hope that both of my girls get such a magical day, surrounded by those who love them, embracing birth and truly enjoying the experience.

**Mama**
Elizabeth Eilers Sullivan

**Baby**
Peter William ("Liam")
born February 4 at 11:24 a.m.
8 pounds 3 ounces
20 inches

# I Am Not a Patient

My labor nurse calls out, "Soon, there will be two patients." What does she mean? Her statement takes me out of my focus, away from my body, away from my baby boy—this "patient" she's talking about—and out to the sterile instruments sparkling in the winter sunlight that streams through the hospital window.

My resolve comes flooding back to me: I am not meant to sit idle in bed, awaiting Liam's arrival. I do not want to be drugged and disconnected from this experience, this new little life. I've done that before. I've been a patient before. But not today.

Today, we are meant to be a team. Our job—one shared by me, Liam, and even our doctor and nurses—is to create a safe and sacred space for birth to happen in its own time. No need for inter*fear*ing, no need to stand on high alert, no need to alter this blessed process.

I bring my awareness back to Liam. Present to each moment, I coax this child out of my womb, listening to what my body and my baby have to say with each rush. Liam is active, strong, and intricately moving, laboring with me to be born. I'm confident in my body's natural ability and my baby's natural wisdom.

*I am not a patient.*

I need a little time to get in the right position to help my baby find his way into the world, and I am painfully aware at every moment how anxious my doctor is as I do this. Liam's heartbeat is steady, sweet, and strong, stronger than the distraction of the nurse fretting over the fetal monitor. I stand tall. I won't lie down! I swivel my hips. I call on Mother Nature's gift of gravity to help Liam move forward. He and I, we ebb and flow with the natural rhythms of birth, like waves creating the shore.

*I am not a patient.*

Liam takes his time coming down the birth canal. I focus, searching for the right position, the right movement. My doctor, unable to help and more accustomed to being in charge of her patients, begins to chat about the trouble with her garage door this morning. What?! I come out of my zone long enough to command, "Doctor, focus!" Doesn't she realize what's going on in this room? Does she not find birth miraculous?

The nurse continues to fuss with the fetal monitor. To find my boy's heartbeat—and to reassure the nurse—I needed to put the fetal heartbeat monitor on the wall of my vagina. Liam had moved so far down that the nurse was no longer in tune with my child. But I was.

I push for two hours, pushing like I pushed with my first beautiful baby. Fear seizes me, and I wonder whether I'm going to have to expend my precious birthing energy fighting off threats of a vacuum extraction, like I did last time. Then, in the middle of a push, I realize that that's the very thing holding me back, holding Liam back—this fear of the vacuum. Free of the heavy epidural I'd accepted last time, this time I focus on the pressure of Liam's head. I feel the strength of my own legs. I feel my baby beginning to emerge.

*I am not a patient. Liam is not a patient.*

He comes into the world calm, content, tired, a little blue. But I can feel his steady breath, ever so sweetly on my skin, this soft and subtle new breath, consistent and flowing. I guard Liam from the nurse's habit of wiping the afterbirth from baby's skin with that rough, dimpled blue hospital paper. I savor his sweet "newness" on my sweaty body, cherishing our first embrace as mother and son.

Despite what the hospital bracelet suggests, I am not a patient. I am a mother, a wise woman. I am one strong mama.

Erika Rasmusson Janes

**Baby**
Jackson
born October 22 at 12:37 p.m.
6 pounds 15 ounces
19 inches

# Birth Is What It Is

**Before I got pregnant, I** had a passing interest in all things eco-friendly. I recycled my magazines, newspapers, and Diet Coke cans, and ate organic when it was convenient. I admired a friend who composted, but I wasn't ready to do it myself.

Fast-forward to my pregnancy: I was careful (read: neurotic) about what I ate. I relegated house cleaning to my husband, so as not to ingest anything with even a whiff of toxicity. I spent hours researching organic baby gear. I bought cloth diapers. Adding natural childbirth to my Earth Mama list seemed like a no-brainer.

Except that it wasn't. My husband and I attended natural childbirth class, and while I liked much of what I learned, I couldn't quite define why it was important to me. I don't turn down Novocain at the dentist, so why turn down pain medication in the delivery room? Quite simply, my inner Earth Mama wanted to experience the yin and yang of childbirth, the pain and the glory. I knew there could be satisfaction gained from pushing my body beyond what I thought possible.

I told anyone who asked that I was "hoping" for a natural childbirth but wasn't ruling out an epidural. I tried to be prepared for—and open to—whatever experience I might have. I didn't want to set my heart on a natural childbirth, only to need a Cesarean section. I didn't want to feel like a failure if I cried out for an epidural. I *did* want my baby to be born in the way that was best for him.

Apparently, that was at thirty-seven weeks. *Saturday Night Live* ended, but my night was just beginning. My water broke in a slow, incontinent trickle, so I put on a maxi pad and told myself it was false labor. It was not.

Hours passed. Contractions were timed. Deep, low moans were emitted (was that really me mooing and hanging over the back of the couch?). I remembered what my favorite prenatal yoga instructor had told me: *Open throat, open vagina.* I softened my jaw and shoulders, and tried to relax as much as possible into the contractions. My husband massaged my back and waited for the signs of the different stages of labor. More hours passed. I abandoned my bathrobe and paced around the house naked. Finally, we called our doula—and a cab.

At the hospital, I felt sure I'd be sent away. Three centimeters? Four? It had only been eight hours since that trickle. I thought, This is going to go on and on, and I won't be able to bear it. Happily, I was 8 centimeters dilated and my boy's head was visible. Let's have a baby!

Soon I was at 10 centimeters, ready to push. But I didn't feel ready. There was no unbearable urge to expel my baby. I pushed anyway. And pushed, and pushed, and pushed. My doula wiped my chest and brow, and offered me sips of juice while my husband, bless him, held a leg and provided resistance—and encouragement—for each seemingly endless push.

I'm not a religious person, but I prayed. I fingered a ring that contained my late father's birthstone and asked him for strength. *Please don't let me need a C-section now.* Then a mantra came to me: *It is what it is.* My labor is what it is, and my boy will be born how he's supposed to be born. That mantra sustained me through those final burning pushes, until the moment of immeasurable, whooshing relief, and the joy of warm, tiny, baby Jackson being placed on my chest.

I'm in awe of my body. I'm thrilled that I had a natural childbirth, and I'm grateful for whatever role luck and good birthing hips might've played. I hope to satisfy my inner Earth Mama with another natural birth one day. And if I do, I'll remain open-minded, because birth is what it is.

**Mama**

Patty Born Selly

**Baby**

Lucia Rose (Lucy)

born July 29 at 10:30 a.m.

7 pounds .2 ounces

19 inches

# Peaceful, Beautiful Birth

**Birth is phenomenal! Because I** was really, really nervous about birthing, I learned HypnoBirthing® comfort measures to prepare for labor. I labored at home for as long as possible with my husband and my doula. And when it was time to go to the hospital, I "just knew" it was time, as everyone had promised me I would!

When we got to the hospital, I labored there just long enough for the birthing tub to be filled. I climbed in, pushed for twenty minutes or so, and out came my beautiful daughter Lucy. She looked instantly familiar to me. Her birth was very peaceful, very beautiful, and completely awe-inspiring. I was surprised to learn that labor was totally manageable, and I actually felt strong in the face of the challenge, just letting my body do the work. For months afterward, I felt high as a kite!

With Lucy's birth and with the birth of my second baby, Julian, I was completely in awe of myself as a woman, and totally reverent of mothers everywhere. Birth is such a miracle! Childbirth and motherhood have turned me inside out in so many ways. I feel like I've become a newborn: learning as I go, figuring out this new world of children, and parenting, and raising a family.

**Mama**
Mery Vargas Mares

**Baby**
Mateo Daniel
born August 12 at 6:22 a.m.
7 pounds 5 ounces
19½ inches

# Happy Birthday, Baby!

**From the instant the doctor** first told me that my baby's due date was August 5—and later when it changed to August 9—I knew that I would give birth on *my* birthday, August 12. I was also convinced I'd be having a boy, but I waited to share that bit of intuition until he arrived.

Sure enough, I went over my due date, and the morning of the eve of my twenty-sixth birthday, I turned to my husband as we woke and said, "I'm going into labor tonight, and having the baby tomorrow morning." I was so calm and in a state of pure joy all day. I practiced my deep yoga breath all day, and when I went into labor that night, I did my favorite yoga poses.

Before I knew it, we were in the car heading to the hospital. At about 4 a.m., a contraction sent a powerful vibe through my body. My head jerked up, and my eyes alit on a fire dancing in the northwest sky. How fitting and inspiring, I thought! August is the month of Leo, and fire is the main element for my star sign. I felt for sure my boy would be as passionate and as fiery as the blaze that accompanied his birth in the dark of the early morning—a true Leo!

Arriving at the hospital, I was 8 centimeters dilated. I refused an IV and drugs. I wanted to feel the womanly power of going to the absolute edge, persevering, and conquering that edge. When I was fully dilated, I asked to use the squat bar to help me push. My doula and my nurse set it up, although the nurse had never seen one used and they had to search for it! My focus was so intense. I was completely in the moment. I asked to have a mirror in front of me so I could see my baby emerge.

I would squat as I pushed, and then stand up on the hospital bed to shake my legs out between pushes. I have never felt such intensity and power possessing my body. I was exhausted, yet something inside me kept me going. I reached that edge I'd hoped to conquer, and at 6:22 a.m., our baby boy was born.

When we saw him, we chose the name we saw in his face: Mateo Daniel. In Spanish, *Mateo* means "gift from God." And on that blazing hot August night, with the delivery room full of earthshaking womanly power and love, God did just that. He sent me the greatest birthday gift ever!

**Mama**
Catherine Burns

**Babies**
Erin
born March 14 at 1:42 p.m.
6 pounds 4 ounces
19 inches

Lee
born September 11 at 1:30 p.m.
7 pounds
19½ inches

# She'll Be Coming Around the Mountain

**The births of each of** my children were intense and inspiring events. I labored at home as long as possible, where I could move in comfort and safety with my husband and childbirth assistants. At each birth we arrived at the hospital elevators coming into transition. Just what I wanted; no time for interventions. In the room it all came down to me and my baby, with my assistants in the background. My helpers allowed me to go into myself deeply and just track with whatever I needed. At Erin's birth, my first child, we paused before the final crowning push. Out of the blue spring sky I sang, all verses:

*She'll be coming around the mountain when she comes*
*She'll be driving six white horses when she comes*
*We'll all be here to meet her when she comes*
*We'll all be glad to see her when she comes*

So clearly, I have the image of Erin coming around and through the bony passes of my pelvis, powerfully moving into the opening.

With my second, Lee, I could feel him dropping through the pelvic bones, separating them incrementally. What a way to experience intensity! Instead of feeling it as pain, I thought, This is my baby opening my bones because *he* is moving down. He let me know exactly where we were in labor!

Each of my babies arrived bright eyed and pinking up; I was euphoric and shaking; each one was a gift to the world.

I was deeply supported in my pregnancies and births by somatic therapy. These mind-body movement and mindfulness practices provided grounding into myself and trust in the natural process of my own rhythms. After Erin was born, I felt strongly that other women should have the chance to prepare for birth in this way. Her birth compelled me to create MamaBebe, a prenatal class for natural birth preparation. Lo and behold, within one week of sending out a mailing, I was pregnant with Lee. I got to teach my first class for myself and two other women.

For women, birth instills in us the feminine power of creation and prepares us to be mother bears for our children. For our babies, the birth experience imprints the ability to initiate, follow through, fulfill, and complete activities.

The great gift of my births has been the steadfast conviction and courage in handling both the normal challenges and the intense curveballs that life throws us. I am deeply grateful for the beautiful and satisfying work— which has evolved to include developmental playgroups, training for early childhood staff, developmental movement therapy for children with autism spectrum disorders, and more—that my children have led me to undertake.

**Mama**
Jennifer Tacheny

**Baby**
Delvin Thomas
born September 19 at 5:08 a.m.
7 pounds 7 ounces
20 inches

# Keep Singing to Me

**Monday, September 18, I worked** late. I'd felt light contractions throughout the day, but there was no pain. I recall feeling *big* that evening. I told a colleague I felt full and large.

9:30 p.m.
I head home and take a bath.

10:30 p.m.
In bed.

12:45 a.m.
Mild menstrual-like cramps in my low belly wake me. I walk around, do some laundry, sit in the nursery rocking chair.

1:10 a.m.
My husband, Steven, awakes to find me walking about. We agree that the cramps are probably Braxton Hicks. But we do call the midwife—Jennifer is on-call—because I have a touch of bleeding. She thinks I'm in early labor and says to get some sleep. The ache in my belly worsens when I lie down. I get up and hear a light *pop,* my water breaking.

1:30 a.m.
I call Jennifer back to say I'm definitely in labor. We decide that I'll take a warm bath and call her when things pick up. I soak for thirty minutes. The crampy feelings continue.

2 a.m.
Once I'm out of the bath, things change dramatically. The contractions are much stronger, and I get about thirty

seconds between each surge of pain. Steven calls his mom. I'm focused and efficient, throwing last-minute items into my hospital bag, stopping during each contraction to hold steady against the bedroom door frame, grounding through the intensity.

My moans turn to wails as I try to breathe through the pain. Steven, finishing last-minute lesson plans for his substitute teacher, calls up from the main level, "Keep singing to me." I don't have the heart—or the ability—to say I'm not exactly singing.

2:30 a.m.
Steven calls the midwife to say we're headed for the hospital. Right now!

3 a.m.
Mom arrives just in time for us to leave the house. I'm gripping the stair post, struggling through another contraction. Mom, who has birthed six children, motions to Steven that we have no time to waste.

We run red lights all the way to the hospital. The ride to the hospital feels like one LONG, HARD contraction.

3:30 a.m.
Hospital. At last!

Mom presses the emergency call button. "We have a woman in labor here!" she says. A security guard fetches a wheelchair in what felt like slow motion. I choose to walk.

As we head toward the birthing room, I start shedding my clothes, and I strip entirely the instant we arrive. A squatting position on the bed suits my pain. A nurse quickly checks the baby's heart rate and inserts an antibiotic IV to protect my baby from Strep B.

"Midwife. Need midwife!" I demand, and the nurse tells me Jennifer is on her way—from Wisconsin, some thirty miles away. "Wisconsin!" I cry in disbelief. Then I dive into the next contraction.

As I lean into Steven and Mom, I feel the need to push, and my body bears down. When that contraction ends, I see our midwife arriving, looking every bit the country midwife: unwrapping her hand-knit scarf from her neck, untying her wool sweater from her waist, red clogs that remind me of my own black pair. I'm relieved that she's here, and that she seems more like me than not.

The midwife's first move is most graceful. She positions herself in front of me and places her hands gently on my forehead as I bear forward. Then she puts her forehead against mine and says, "That's right, on the next contraction push again just like you did on the last one."

4:30 a.m.
I push through five more long contractions, three enduring pushes each time, swaying my hips back and forth.

"Your body knows what to do. That's right, sway your hips and move that baby down the birth canal," my midwife instructs. I feel like my body, my instincts, are leading the way. Then Jennifer directs me into a sitting position and has me lower the tone of my moans; both changes encourage the baby to move down the canal, she says.

For a few contractions, we all—Mom, Steven, Jennifer, me—moan in chorus. Then I need silence: "SHHH, no talking." There is only my moaning roar and Zen chanting "zoo, zoo, za, za, zee, zee." This is the most amazing moment in labor. Hope and focus fill the early-morning, dimly lit room.

"I can see your baby," Jennifer says. Mom and Steven take a peek, and then I grab their arms and demand they stay right next to me for the final few contractions.

5:08 a.m.
Our baby boy is born!

I reach down between my thighs and pull him to my chest. "It's a boy! My beautiful baby, my beautiful baby, my beautiful baby!" I exclaim. He gives a little cry and breathes his first breath while lying on my chest. The scent of this new life   maple syrup, black licorice   fills the room and swells its way into my memory forever. Steven cuts the umbilical cord, and we relax, savoring those first minutes of life with our son, Delvin Thomas.

Mama
Delina Codey

**Baby**
Teo
born September 25 at 5:14 p.m.
8 pounds 13 ounces
21 inches

# Becoming a Mother

**The contraction woke me at** 12:30 a.m., seizing my lower back like a menstrual cramp on steroids, fierce enough that I had to remind myself to keep breathing. After weeks of worrying—when will it start? what if I'm in public? what if I don't make it to the hospital in time?—my labor had begun.

Ten minutes apart, one minute in duration, exactly how the birthing class had promised. I timed my contractions alone, slowly counting, slowly breathing, hoping between each one for sleep.

I could have awoken my husband, and he would have sat with me in nervous excitement, timing contractions, rubbing my back, bringing me water, offering ice cream. Instead, I left him in bed and crept to the living room. I wanted him rested, but more than that, I wanted to await the dawn alone, to hold close the final moments when my life was all my own.

Rocking, contracting, I watched the sky lighten, from black to indigo, to the curious pale green of dawn. Soon, it was time to wake my husband, to call the doctor, to call my parents, to invite the world into the birth of this child.

In the elevator, on the sidewalk, people looked from me to my husband, to our stack of suitcases and the telltale car seat. They smiled and wished us luck. Our Sikh cabdriver talked reverently about the joy of children, and drove us as close to the hospital entrance as he could without crashing through the lobby.

I spent the first few hours in the birthing center walking the hallways, bending over to breathe as each contraction built, then continuing on my laps and chatting with the nurses. I was proud of how I was handling my labor, sure that I'd be delivering this baby with grace and ease. What was all the talk of unbearable pain, the need for epidurals? Then, my doctor examined me and found that I was 7 centimeters, just 1 centimeter more than I'd been three hours earlier.

"I can break your water," my OB said. "It will probably speed this up a bit." I was, in theory, against birth interventions, but I was getting tired of all the walking, all the chatting. I was here, I was ready. Why not?

My water breaking was strangely soothing, but very quickly I realized that my graceful labor was over. As my son's head ground down into my cervix, I shuffled in tight circles between the bed and the wall, forcing motion against the pain that reared bright red and blinding. Despite years as a distance runner and months of daily swimming, the ten feet in my room was almost more than I could manage.

I soon sank into the tub and held on. I bobbled and kicked. My husband, soaking wet, leaned over to rub my back. Being held weightless lessened the pain, and when I moaned, screamed, and groaned, the water absorbed my cries. Eventually, a shuddering took hold. It was time to push.

With each new contraction I took a deep breath and bore down, twice, three times, before falling back into a relaxation as deep as sleep. Washcloths on my forehead, a straw with Gatorade in my mouth, encouraging words, a mirror wheeled in. I looked at the tiny, quarter-sized bit of head emerging, vanishing, appearing again, and tried not to think about how many more pushes remained.

The quarter became a lime, an orange, a grapefruit—all the stages of fetal growth repeated as my son's head descended. And then, those magical words, "One more push, and the head is out." The last push is the fiercest. It's the moment we hold as mothers, the moment our child is born. I summoned a courage I had not known, a determination to meet my child. One more push, through a ring of fire.

After this, we can endure anything—even labor, again. Everyone says women forget the pain of childbirth, that that's the only reason we go and get pregnant again. I don't think that's quite it. I think we can remember the pain if we want to, but more than that, we remember the tangle of limbs in our arms, the wide-open eyes, slate blue, searching for Mama. This is why we have children. When they lie in sleep across our chests, we are reminded of tiny elbows, of ankles under our rib cages. We hold their heads, smooth their sweaty hair, and think, This dear one was inside me, sleeping inside my hip bones. And we want to try this miracle again.

As mothers, we carry always the children who were once within us. We feed them and rock them, kiss them and teach them, bear witness to their discoveries and hold them when they fall. We fight when they need us to and stand back when we must, with the same courage and determination that we summoned to bring them forth. Giving birth is our transformation from women into mothers. And with that, we give birth to a strength and a love we have never known.

Melissa Rayworth

**Baby**
Mason
born June 21 at 12:08 p.m.
7 pounds 7 ounces
18 inches

# Don't Sweat the Small Stuff

In the early spring of 2003, just as my third trimester began, my husband, Ted—a journalist—flew to the Persian Gulf to cover the earliest days of the Iraq War. We were living in China at the time, and the SARS epidemic had begun raging. Doctors were worried about the risk to pregnant women and doubtful about trusting the official reports on the spread of SARS. My doctor in Beijing said he felt sure the government was lying about how fast the illness was spreading, but he could only guess how much was being covered up. That was all Ted and I needed to hear. I flew to Pittsburgh to spend the final months of my pregnancy with my in-laws. We'd planned all along to deliver the baby in the United States, but suddenly I was hurrying there months ahead of schedule.

As the weeks progressed and my Braxton Hicks contractions intensified, it became clear that my first responsibility to my unborn son was to remain as calm and positive and strong as I possibly could.

Ted managed to call on the satellite phone once a day, even if it meant lying down on the rooftop of his Baghdad hotel to avoid gunfire. We stayed connected despite the thousands of miles between us. I watched CNN obsessively, as though keeping tabs on the war would somehow help keep Ted safe. In my first trimester, I'd wondered how I'd manage the job of being someone's mother. Now at the end of my pregnancy, as the days crawled by, I grew confident in my ability to take care of this little person. There was no time for doubting myself. I had to stay focused on carrying this baby to full term.

I had only seen my son's grainy image on the ultrasound, but I felt as if I knew him already. Mason and I lay awake together through long nights spent hoping Ted would come home safely, choosing to believe that he would. Mason would roll around in my belly and I would tell him when my fear threatened to get the best of me. I'd promise him I wouldn't let it bring tears, or contractions. Sometimes, I'd say it out loud.

Early on, Mason helped me learn the most useful skill a mother can have: not to sweat the small stuff. Amid the obvious concerns of whether my husband would make it home to meet his son, and whether my son would make it to thirty-seven weeks, other upsets seemed minor. Like the time my house sitter in Beijing called to say that the children of NBA player Wang Zhizhi, who lived upstairs, had flooded their apartment and, subsequently, mine.

"Don't worry," I told my house sitter. "It's only water."

There was silence, then:

"The plaster walls are kind of melting," he said, "and I don't know what's gonna happen to your stuff. How come you're not freaking out? You usually, you know . . . freak out over stuff like that."

The answer was simple. "Ted is alive, or at least he was an hour ago when he called, and Mason is still in my belly at thirty-five weeks. If both of them are healthy and unharmed, I'm not going to freak out over a flooded apartment." (I must confess, though, that I asked him to move all my favorite shoes to higher ground; a girl's gotta draw the line somewhere.)

On June 14, as week thirty-seven began, Ted returned from Baghdad as promised. Six days later, I went into labor.

Labor—I'd been so worried about how I'd handle it. But when we finally found ourselves in the delivery room, I trusted that Mason and I would find our way, just as we had through that last trimester. It was as if the three of us were already a family, pulling together to accomplish something. (Six hours into laboring, I did beg for and get an epidural. I'd had my fill of positive thinking by that point.)

When the nurse put my boy in my arms six hours later, it was more like a reunion than an introduction. We'd been there for each other through three strange, uncertain, and ultimately life-changing months. Suddenly, the days ahead seemed far more manageable.

Mama

Laura Stoland

**Baby**

Siri

born May 11 at 11:25 a.m.

7 pounds 9 ounces

19½ inches

# From in Me to on Me

**"I think I might be** in labor," I answer when Deidre, the owner of Perch, our local coffee shop, asks me how I'm doing. It's Thursday morning and I'm attending a sing-along with Jack, my sixteen-month-old son. My membranes had been stripped the day before, and things feel, well, strange. But the so-called 5/1/1—contractions five minutes apart lasting for one minute for one hour—isn't happening.

By nighttime I'm getting excited, but I don't want to wake my doctor with a false alarm. I'm concerned about the logistics of leaving Jack in the middle of the night. I decide to wait and see what happens next. Jack was induced, so I'm savoring the natural beginning of labor. The pain is intensifying, but I manage it by walking the upstairs hallway and sitting on the toilet. I feel ready for this adventure.

I fall asleep and wake up a few times during the night, thinking I can't possibly be in labor if I'm sleeping through it. By 5:30 a.m., still no regular contractions to track. But the pain is so present that I begin to wonder how I'll endure the car ride. I call Dr. Russell. "Take your time, shower, eat something, and I'll meet you at the hospital," she says. Excited and happy, Ira, my husband, calls the neighbor to come over for Jack. I finish packing, kiss sleeping Jack, and we leave.

The car ride is tough. Without being able to move around as I wish, it's hard to make it through the contractions. Finally, I check into the hospital and soon learn that I'm 7 centimeters dilated. Well, that seems manageable! If I'm already that far along I should be able to make it through the whole thing without drugs, right? Little did I know what opening my body those last 3 centimeters would take.

Dirty bathroom, no hot water for a shower, IV in my arm, yucky thin sheets, metal railing on the bed, cold tile floor—I hate hospitals. The happy progress I had made through the night seems to disappear.

But I soon find it again, leaning on Ira, half standing with my arms around his neck and my eyes closed while Kenzie, my doula, rubs my lower back hard. The rhythm in the pain, the rest between the contractions. Anchored to Ira, the pain is bearable. We are riding it, working through it, opening my body slowly, painfully but willingly for this new little person we are so excited to meet. Periodically, the nurses come in and make me lie on the bed with the fetal monitor on. Those moments are almost unbearable. Without Ira's body against mine, I am lost in a sea of pain.

It can't get any worse than this, right? It can't go on much longer, right? Wrong. And wrong again.

On my side, exhausted, moaning like an animal. So intense I can't even see. The world is a swirl of blasting spots before my eyes. I can't think, talk, or move other than to try to escape this pain beyond pain. If it were possible to get an epidural now, I would gladly put the needle in myself. It's not. I'm way too far along.

I—am—being—ripped—apart—at—my—core.

Dr. Russell says the baby is ready to come anytime I am ready to push her out. I don't feel capable. Dr. Russell picks my leg up and bends it to help me push; I feel I have no control over my body.

Then, she's crushing, squeezing, sliding out.

Siri is here!

As intensely as the pain rocked my every cell, it is suddenly and completely gone, replaced by tearful bliss.

I'm so proud of both of us for making this journey.

From in me to on me. To the breast!

Lovely. Alert. Hungry!

Perfect.

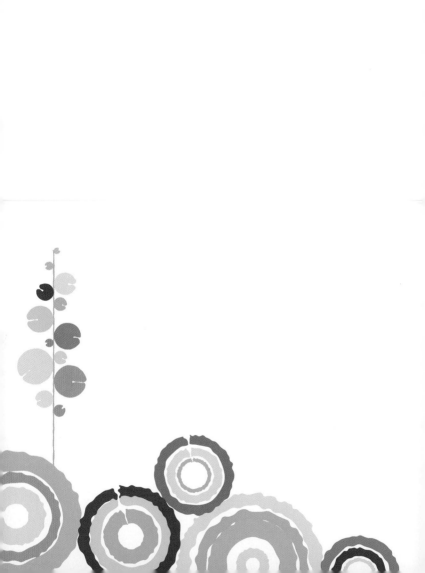

# Home Births

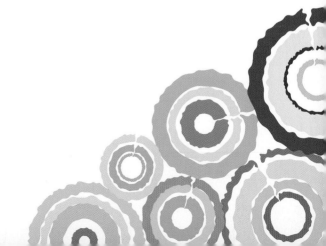

**Mama**
Barb Haselbeck

**Baby**
Alexandra
born April 20 at 9 a.m.
Little sister to Chris
born November 14 at 2:30 a.m.

# The Nature of Birth

**In the darkness of an** April night, deep muscular twinges awake me after a few hours of sleep. That evening we had feasted with friends on lasagna, salad, garlic bread, and sweet-tart lemon pie—all homemade. I had eaten heartily, somehow making room for the meal in a stomach that had less room than usual as neighbor to my nine-months-pregnant womb. Now I shift to my other side, sure that I recognize the ache of early labor, but waiting, wanting to be sure before I wake up my husband, John. I harbor within myself the knowledge that birthing has begun, savoring it before telling anyone else, having to make preparations, or phone my midwife.

Fully alert within five minutes, I wait another ten and nudge John. Hearing the news, he awakes even more quickly than I had. With our firstborn, Chris, he alternately read the Bible and smoked cigarettes in the living room while two angelic midwives ministered to me, applying hot compresses to my belly and massaging my limbs, absorbing and dispersing my tension. Though an awkward labor coach, John was at my side much of the time. His presence and arms provided tremendous support.

Now, we quickly perform our morning rituals so we can prepare the birthing bed. First we move our sleeping son from our queen-sized family bed to another room, then outfit the bed with a clean bottom sheet, a plastic sheet, and a final layer of sterile sheet. My contractions are fifteen minutes apart. Time to call my midwife, Leigh, who lives about fifty-five miles south of us. We are living in the Chequamegon National Forest in northwestern Wisconsin. Our house sits on a three-hundred-acre estate, where John is the property manager. Our nearest neighbor is five miles to the east, the nearest town fourteen miles west, and nearest hospital thirty miles. It's now about 3:30 a.m. Leigh sounds sleepy and suggests I call when the contractions are ten minutes apart. John decides to take a walk around the smaller lake on the property. This makes me uneasy, even though I know it will take only about twenty minutes. My previous labor lasted twelve hours, so there should be plenty of time. Chris is sleeping soundly, with no idea that this is his last day as an only child. I walk around, eat a little yogurt, think I feel pressure on my cervix. My sense of well-being and anticipation makes me alert.

By the time John returns, contractions are ten minutes apart. I feel pleased at this steady progress as I call Leigh; still sleepy, she suggests I call her back when they are five minutes apart! I think this is a bit strange, but I'm not too worried. When I mention the pressure I feel within and that the midwife has not left yet, it's too much—John calls our dinner friends, who had given birth at home just three months earlier. Fortunately, they have stayed overnight in a nearby cabin.

For the third time, I called Leigh. Night was lifting, and the sun rested just below the horizon.

"Things are moving right along. My contractions are five minutes apart."

"OK, I'm leaving right now," she says. Later, when I find out she is three months pregnant, I remember how one sleeps at that stage—intoxicated with the need for it, day or night.

I decide to walk outside in the fresh air as I had with my first labor, before the intensity of labor forces me to lie down. Leaning into John, we walk slowly down the first slope of a high hill on which our log house sits. We pass the bird feeder, sitting above the berry bushes. At the foot of the slope, I turn to look back at the house and the large window that faces the lake.

"Wait." I need to slow down, to pause for the wave of pain that clenches inside me. I know when I return indoors I will be heading for the bed. The mild April air refreshes and gently draws me away from my inner focus. The sun's first rays halo the trees but have not yet hit the dark ice on the lake.

John is sitting at my bedside when a contraction breaks the amniotic sac so forcefully that it showers him in a spray of fluid. Otherwise, my labor is textbook. At 9 a.m., my daughter, Alexandra, is born into bright sunshine that streams into the bedroom. The nature of her arrival is in keeping with her own intense personality. She protests with full lung capacity the light, brilliant to eyes accustomed to muted shades of darkness.

Leigh had arrived at 7:30, just as I entered the pushing stage. Now she says, "Look how pretty she is." Still in a daze, I say stupidly, "She is?" Shortly after Alexandra's birth, several friends have arrived. We are startled to hear a loon call out, the first of the year, a true sign of spring. According to woods lore, the return of the loons heralds the breakup of the ice. On that day, April 20, 1980, the temperature reaches 80 degrees; no trace of ice is left on the lake.

Mama
Bridget Foley

**Baby**
Liam Nelson
born April 29 at 12:59 a.m.
7 pounds 15 ounces
21 inches

# Sacred Ceremony

**After years of witnessing other** women bring babies into the world as a doula, I wanted my birth time to be a sacred ceremony. So I chose to birth at home, with midwives and a birth coach.

On April 28, one week past our "guess date," I was on my yoga mat, rolling around on my exercise ball. I'd had some contractions, and I was anxious to get things under way. Suddenly I heard a loud *pop*—and my water broke, gushing all over the yoga mat.

I called my dear yoga teacher, Ana Forrest, and spoke with her as I waited for my "team" to arrive. When my midwives checked me, I was 3 centimeters dilated and completely effaced. My birth coach, Kathy, arrived. I felt truly ready to birth once I saw her. I was using the Hypnobabies® techniques she had taught. The hypnosis was supposed to help me feel pressure instead of pain, but I felt pain—lots and lots of pain!

I labored nine more hours. Kathy talked me through every contraction, reminding me of cues to help me manage the sensations. Her counterpressure on my lower back opened my pelvis and eased the discomfort.

We had a kiddie pool set up in our bedroom, and I spent a lot of time in there. I also sat on the exercise ball and the toilet, squatted, and got on my hands and knees. The one position that didn't work was lying on my side. I needed to move the energy out of my pelvis and down through my feet into the floor.

In addition to the professionals, I had the support of my husband, William, who was incredible; our friends Dianna and Matthew, who became Liam's godparents; and Beatriz, a photographer who shot the birth. It was a large "staff," but I needed all of them. Aside from their appointed roles, they formed a bucket brigade to keep the pool water warm. Our midwives told us they'd never been at a birth with such incredible energy; I had a special bond with everyone there, and that eased the process for me.

By 9 p.m. I had to make a choice. I'd dilated to 6 centimeters. The intensity had grown, and I needed to adopt a better attitude. I was thinking I'd been an idiot to try birthing naturally at home, and I was convinced I never wanted to have another baby. If I'd been in a hospital, I would have begged for an epidural. I considered asking to transfer to a hospital, but the thought of having contractions in the car en route felt inconceivable. I gave myself a stern internal talking-to and decided I could keep going. Later, everyone said I appeared really calm. I had them fooled!

Around 11 p.m. one of my midwives had me bear down while she rimmed my cervix. In one contraction I reached 10 centimeters, ready to push. I'd hoped that once I reached the pushing stage I'd feel more pressure and less pain—instead I felt pressure *and* pain! It turned out that Liam's arms were pinned alongside his face. He came into the world Superman fashion, or like Edvard Munch's *The Scream*, one hand over his ear, the other alongside his chin.

I pushed well, but it took two hours to deliver him. My midwife had to hold Liam's arms in close by his head so that he wouldn't wing out an elbow and lacerate my tender parts. To her great credit, I came through with one tiny tear, too small for her even to stitch.

I was on the bed pushing (clutching the headboard and screeching like some prehistoric bird) when Liam crowned. I looked at William, standing at the foot of our bed alongside the midwife. We locked eyes. I pushed with the next contraction and Liam's head and arms emerged, followed by the rest of his sweet self. They laid him on my belly. A profound hush came over us all in the dim light (it was 12:59 a.m.). Liam looked around, alert and curious. He yawned a few times as I held him, William's hand on his back. We stayed that way for a long while.

Since his first moments in the world, Liam has been a sweet boy. We feel so blessed and lucky to have him. And while I swore during labor that I'd never go through that again, now I feel empowered. Liam's about to turn one, and William and I are talking about starting on our next collaborative endeavor—a brother or sister for our little boy bundle of joy.

**Mama**
Anne Bachhuber

**Baby**
Sylvan Renate
born April 29 at 7:31 p.m.
7 pounds
20 inches

# Full Moon Rising

I lived on a commune, East Wind Community, in the Missouri Ozarks when I birthed my daughter, Sylvan. The culture there was dramatically different from the mainstream. Mamas breast-fed as long as they wanted to, nearly everyone followed the tenets of attachment parenting, and pretty much every mom had a home birth with a midwife. I was no exception: I chose a midwife who came highly recommended by several other moms. Because of the rural setting, it was a long drive to meet her for prenatal visits, but we made the two-and-a-half-hour trip often.

Not long after I learned I was pregnant, I dreamt that I would give birth on April 29, and I stubbornly clung to that idea for my entire pregnancy. I even had my mom come out a couple of days early so that she wouldn't miss it. On the 29th, I woke up at 5 a.m., feeling like, "OK, I'm ready." And, of course, nothing happened.

For hours and hours (and hours), I kept waiting to go into labor, but nothing. Finally, I gave up, lay down for a nap, and couldn't sleep.

Then around 5 p.m., my bag of waters started leaking, just a trickle. I woke my partner, Sorrel, and we waited to see what would happen. Within fifteen minutes, I went from mild, squeezy contractions to full-on intense, crazy Technicolor ones. I remember thinking, I have thirteen more hours of this?!? I also remember thinking that the contractions felt nothing like the belly squeeze I had expected. They felt low and grinding and pressure-filled.

Sorrel set up a blanket and a big body pillow outside in the sun so that I could relax and try to pull it together for the next thirteen hours I imagined I'd be in labor. My mom came to our cabin, which was down the hill a ways from the rest of the community. A couple of women, Sarah and Ivy, came to help while we waited for the midwife.

Somewhere around 6:15, I started feeling the urge to push. My mom, a nurse, had me pant and pant and try not to push, because I was obviously just starting what we all expected to be a stereotypically long labor. Finally, I couldn't hold back anymore. I pushed and pushed on all fours on that blanket in the sun. I had a lot of back labor, meaning my daughter likely wasn't in quite the right position. But Sorrel pressed on my spine while my mom cheered me on and held my head in her lap. Sarah sat behind me, ready to catch the baby if necessary, and Ivy boiled water, took pictures, and did whatever else needed doing.

At 7:31 p.m., just two and a half hours after my labor started, I gave birth to my daughter. The sun was setting and the full moon rising. The pictures from that day are beautiful, with everyone backlit by the sun in the tall grass, with incongruous medical supplies—sent by my dad, a doctor—littering the ground. An hour later, the midwife arrived, complimented Sarah on a job well done, looked me over, and called it a day.

Ten years later, I'm a nursing student. I recently completed my obstetrics clinical rotation. Going from my birth experience to the highly medicalized induction-epidural-Cesarean section version of the birth process was kind of like wandering into a sci-fi dystopic world from a sunshine, happy one. Talk about mind-blowing!

**Mama**
Nicole Roth

**Baby**
Madeline
born January 20 around 2:30 p.m.
10 pounds 5 ounces
22 inches

# Confidence, Richly Rewarded

**For months my husband, Dave,** and I had been collecting items for our home birth. A couple of days past my due date, it was finally time to find out how our midwives, Susan and Angela, planned to use the salt, the garlic, the Crock-Pot, and the washcloths.

Angela went to work preparing the herbal bath mixture, adding the garlic and salt. The Crock-Pot went in the bathroom to warm the washcloths that would be my hot compresses during labor. On the stove, a pot of boiling water sterilized the metal birth instruments. That's when it hit me: I am having a baby! At home. *Today.* Wow!

Having been in active labor for several hours, I was curious about how far along I was. Angela, still a midwifery student, had a hard time finding my cervix, so Susan tried. It was *waaay* back. Ouch! But I was dilated to 5 centimeters. That was encouraging!

As contractions progressed, I swayed with Dave. I'd pull him closer, and he'd move away—freaked out by our baby's strong kicks. The midwives thought that was humorous. I moved to sit on the birthing ball for a bit; Dave sat next to me on the couch, massaging my back.

We dimmed the lights to create a serene atmosphere and listened to the Scripture tape Dave and I had recorded. I had listened to it daily for the past few weeks. What power and promise are in those words! I began to weep. I was struck with a sense of awe and humility as I meditated on the Lord's provision, love, and faithfulness. It felt like a miracle that He brought me to labor strong, prepared, and healed after being so sick just one year earlier, with hypothyroidism, a weakened enlarged heart, breathing problems, and anxiety. Along with faith, a gluten-free diet and a couple of intense healing retreats had restored my health. Susan prayed beautifully while holding my hand, thanking Him for His strong presence and faithfulness. I felt better getting all that emotion out.

I moved to the tub. It felt great; so soothing and relaxing, just like my nightly bath. That's the one time of day I have all to myself, to relax and contemplate.

Time crawled, and I felt discouraged. Susan checked me a few times. I was making progress, but my cervix was still very high. I wondered why it was taking so long.

As the contractions intensified, so did my vocalizations— louder and more guttural. I was surprised those primitive moans came out of me. I think Dave was too! I half-joked that I was in full support of his vasectomy! (Two weeks later, though, I felt ready to do this birth thing all over again!)

Finally, an urge to push. I was complete but had a small lip of cervix, which Susan took care of on the next contraction. That was uncomfortable. After a few pushes, I grew discouraged. I didn't feel strong. I couldn't find a good position. "I don't like this," I said. "I don't like this."

I asked Susan to read the Scripture that the Lord had given me a few weeks earlier. In December, I had been in the hospital with low hemoglobin. Thankfully, it wasn't as bad as we first thought, but my doctor's words stuck in my head: "I don't think a home birth is safe for you." I was battling some fear. The Lord led me to Hebrews 10:35–36: "So do not throw away your confidence; it will be richly rewarded. You need to persevere so that when you have done the will of God, you will receive what he has promised." I went from wavering in doubt and fear to total confidence and peace in a matter of moments.

The water wasn't working anymore, so I slowly moved to the bed. With the next contraction I got on my side, and Angela held my right leg nearly straight up in the air. I felt more powerful.

I pushed for about an hour. I asked for a mirror, as I had when birthing my other two children. I could see some dark hair, and with some hard work over the next couple of contractions, Madeline's head was out. We would soon learn that Madi was a big girl at 10 pounds 5 ounces, which helped explain why the pushing phase lasted so long.

A couple more contractions, and I pushed the rest of Madeline's body out. What an absolute relief! The midwives handed Madi to me, and I snuggled up to her, loving her chubby cheeks and blue eyes. I kept saying, "Oh my gosh, I can't believe it. I can't believe it!" Dave was elated and told me what a great job I did. I felt amazing!

After the cord was cut, we placed Madi on my belly so she could do the "breast crawl" that I had seen in a UNICEF video: Baby crawls from Mama's belly to breast and latches on spontaneously. Madi made the stepping motions on my belly, which helps expel the placenta and prevent hemorrhaging. She stimulated my nipple with her hand and made sucking motions. And then she let us know with her insistent cries that she didn't want to mess around with the breast crawl any longer! We helped her latch on, and she nursed like a champ. Then we got in a healing, cleansing herbal bath. I held Madi so that just her face was out of the water, and we floated for a bit.

Dave had made a great meal of stuffed peppers, but I was too excited and exhausted from the adrenaline rush to do anything but snuggle Madeline, nurse, and revel in the amazing day that we had just experienced. I was not expecting such a long and, at times, difficult labor, but the Lord walked me through each step. Psalm 126:3 says it all: "The LORD has done great things for us, and we are filled with joy."

**Mama**
Heidi Schwinghammer

**Baby**
Gavin
born June 25 at 10:39 a.m.
7 pounds 6 ounces
21 inches

# Gentle Homecoming

I always knew I'd get pregnant right away, when that season of my life arrived.

Fall 2006 was that season. The morning of October 21, I took a pregnancy test. I was already a few weeks pregnant, and I felt I had known it from the day of conception. I had a very powerful dream one night that let me know, and I realized months later that I'd heard the voice of the universe in that dream. Along with the incredible excitement of being pregnant, I was amazed at the belief I had in my inner voice. It was one of those moments in life where I felt I really knew myself and trusted in my self-knowledge.

My pregnancy began about like I expected: a bit of nausea and some exhaustion in the first trimester. After that, I felt pretty well, and I relished my final weeks of pregnancy. I finally had a big belly and couldn't do much because of it. I had six weeks to be pampered, to bask in the kindness of others, to relax and enjoy something I might never experience again.

On Sunday, June 24, at about 3 a.m. I woke up to use the bathroom. When I got back into bed I realized that my water had broken. I excitedly told my husband, we hugged, then finally managed to get back to sleep until about 6 a.m. I felt like cleaning up the house a bit before things really got going. My contractions were ten to fifteen minutes apart and very manageable. I thought to myself, This will be easy if this is what labor is all about! I called my home birth midwives to fill them in, and I realized just how pleased I was that we had chosen to birth at home. No rushing around to pack to get to a hospital.

My contractions seemed to stop, and I decided I'd cleaned the house enough. I knew I needed to relax. My thoughts were centered on being in my own surroundings, in my own home, and with my husband. I went outside with some tea to sit in the warm, comforting late-morning sun. I sat for a few moments in quiet contemplation. Very soon I would be working on bringing a baby into our world.

The contractions picked up again that evening, around 7 p.m. They were more intense and more difficult at three minutes apart. We called the midwives, and as soon as they arrived, I felt relieved and reassured. I got into the nice, hot birthing tub that my husband had spent the day filling and checking. Soothing music filled the room. I couldn't believe how great it felt just being in the tub in the middle of my home. The weightlessness and the warmth of the water really eased my labor. I wished I could have fallen asleep!

I labored through the night and into the next morning. I was in and out of the birthing tub many times. My husband and my midwives took turns applying pressure to my back when a contraction came on. I started pushing around 7:30 a.m. After about an hour, I started to get discouraged, but the midwives said that I was close. I reached down to feel for the baby's head, but I was so tired and concentrating so hard that I didn't feel it at first. I tried again.

There it was! I could feel the crown of my baby's head. I had such a rush of emotion that I started to cry. At the point of exhaustion with my legs freely shaking, feeling my baby for the first time was as comforting as a warm blanket…as though we were encapsulated in a golden ball of light. The reality of a human being—my baby—was real for the first time. I felt we were connected by more than just our bodies; our hearts and souls were connected on a level that I think only a mother can understand.

Our baby was so helpless and fragile as he waited to be born. I just wanted to hold him, to let him know everything was OK. I wanted to kiss him and look into his eyes for the first time. My energy was recharged, and I pushed for another hour and a half. The baby was slowly rocking in the birth canal. We did this back-and-forth for about five hard pushes. I was worried for his head to be in that tight spot for so long. But the midwives assured me that this way was actually easier and gentler for him. That was really all that was important to me: We'd chosen a home birth so that we could have a very gentle and calm experience for this little being, wanting him to enter this world feeling safe and loved, and without intervention or harsh treatment.

I will never forget the moment I first saw Gavin. He was so small and helpless, his body a greenish gray, his head as rippled as sand dunes. He had worked so hard to be born, and now he was in my warm arms. The bump I had been carrying for more than nine months was not just a bump anymore. He was a beautiful baby, opening his eyes for the first time to meet mine with all the love of the universe. Our pregnancy and especially the birth unfolded exactly the way baby Gavin had wanted it to—gently and peacefully.

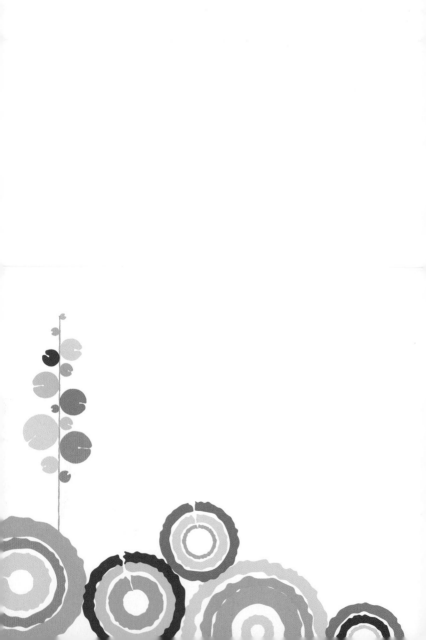

# Extra Special Births

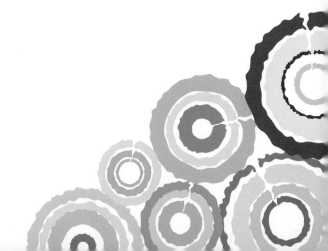

Mama
Kara Douglass Thom

**Babies**
born August 28

McKenna Carolyn at 2:29 p.m.
7 pounds 5 ounces
21¼ inches

Kendall Charlotte at 2:38 p.m.
5 pounds 11 ounces
18 inches

# I Can't Do This!
# I Can Do This!!

**Early in my first pregnancy,** I set my sights on a natural birth. But when I learned at my twenty-week sonogram that I was having twins, I knew my risk for having a Cesarean section increased to greater than 50 percent. Aside from devouring every book I could find about twin pregnancy, I assembled my dream team for birth: an OB who had given birth naturally to twins, an experienced doula, and, of course, my husband.

My pregnancy went so well that at thirty-eight weeks, my cervix was still shut tight. As much as I had hoped to go into labor spontaneously, I knew a scheduled induction was what I faced, raising my anxiety about a Cesarean even higher. My doctor assured me the induction would be slow and gradual and that she would be patient.

I received a dose of Cervidil to soften my cervix at 11 a.m. And then, nothing happened. My husband and I walked, watched movies, and goofed around, all the while wondering when labor would kick in. At 5 p.m., my doctor forced my stubborn cervix to dilate to 1 centimeter and then stripped my membranes. By 10 p.m., we decided to try for a good night's sleep. After tuning off the lights, I rolled over and felt Baby A turn ever so slightly. Suddenly, my water broke. The lights came back on.

Throughout the wee hours of the morning, my husband and our doula helped comfort me as I changed positions on the birthing ball, sat in the rocking chair, and sought relief in the shower. I was having intense back labor, and my doctor and doula worked together to give counterpressure on my hips and help me lunge and squat in hopes of getting Baby A in a better position to move down.

By 5 a.m. I had only progressed to 5 centimeters. I was exhausted. I hadn't slept in twenty-four hours, and I hadn't been back in bed since my water broke. I contemplated the relief an epidural would bring, but I feared it would slow my labor even further. To help with the discomfort of back labor, my doctor administered sterile water injections into my lower back.

Four hours later, I still had not progressed. My doctor felt it was time to enlist the help of Pitocin. In addition, she wanted me to rest. So I got a dose of Nubain, too. It worked: A few hours later I was in transition.

Throughout the night and especially during transition, I heard myself say, "I can't *do* this!" I knew in my head that would be a self-fulfilling prophecy if I repeated it too many times. Sometimes I couldn't help but say it, but as soon as I did, I followed with, "Yes, I can. I can! I *can* do this!"

At last, at 12:30 p.m., I was wheeled into the operating room, just in case either baby needed surgical help. I pushed for two hours before Baby A was born, a girl, weighing 7 pounds 5 ounces. Baby B was transverse, so the nurses tried externally to move her head down. This didn't sit well with Baby B, whose heart rate began to drop. My doctor then tried a breech extraction, but once again, Baby B protested. My doctor couldn't be patient any longer. My doula told me, "Push like your life depends on it!" Once part of the baby's head was showing, and my doctor used the vacuum to expedite her birth. Another little girl came out, a screaming 5 pounds 11 ounces.

It was nothing short of overwhelming joy to have those two healthy babies in my arms. Despite the long, exhausting labor, it was as if the babies were heaven-sent and arrived by magic. I know the real magic was the patience and support I had from my labor team.

**Mama**
Deborah Savran

**Baby**
Gabriel
born February 13 at 7:25 a.m.
7 pounds 7 ounces
20 inches

# Every Birth Is a Rite of Passage

**My path to a planned** Cesarean section was a long journey through grief, toward acceptance, and finally joy. I always wanted a home birth. At the time my children were born, I lived in Australia. The culture there was very much in support of home birth, and I envisioned birthing my babies while gazing serenely through my picture window into the rich rain forest that bordered my home.

But birth wasn't to be that way for me. I had large uterine fibroids that prevented me from experiencing natural childbirth, and learning this was very traumatic for me. I was studying to be a naturopath at the time, so I launched into about a year and a half of desperately trying to heal myself with natural remedies.

Finally, I got a very strong sense that I needed surgery to remove these fibroids—really, to move forward with my life. I've come to think of this as a message from my son, who was waiting to be born. With this surgery, I knew, I would probably never be able to labor naturally because of the scarring on my uterus. Without this surgery, I might never have a child. I found a surgeon I trusted, and he removed the fibroids.

About a year after the surgery, I was pregnant, and I was thrilled! But I had such a strong desire to push this baby out myself. I got second, third, and fourth opinions from doctors and midwives; they all agreed I shouldn't risk labor.

I had a lot of grief about that, and I worked with an energy healer to cope with the loss.

Ultimately, I reached a point of acceptance: If I can't labor, then I will advocate for myself at every point possible, to have the most satisfying birth possible. I wrote the most idyllic Cesarean birth plan. I chose a hospital that agreed to let my baby and me stay together after surgery. Usually, the baby is taken to the nursery until the mother is out of recovery. But I felt strongly that those first moments and hours after birth were immensely important and irreplaceable for the bonding and heart connection between mother and child. This hospital also allowed a midwife to stay with us in the postsurgical recovery room to monitor my health.

By the time we got to the birth day, I was accepting and pretty calm, but somewhat nervous. My husband, David, was with me. I entered the surgery theater on a table, and as they wheeled me into the room, it was filled with light. I could see the angelic nature of all those present and how beautiful everyone was—my husband, my midwife, the doctor, the anesthesiologist, the assistants, the pediatrician. There were eight or nine of us, including me, and I could never have imagined that the environment of that room was going to be what it was. It took my breath away.

I felt everyone was projecting their best qualities; that was all I could see—the pure goodness in everyone who was helping me birth. I was very gushy, very grateful, saying, "Thank you so much for being here, thank you so much for helping!" I remember saying that a lot. It seemed to prompt everyone to give even more of their goodness.

When it was time to deliver my baby, I lay there with the screen protecting the surgical field—and blocking my view. The doctor told me to slow my breathing. I hadn't even realized I was breathing quickly. My husband, standing next to me and watching everything, said, "Here he comes!" as our son, Gabriel, was born. They lifted Gabe up right as he came out, and I remember saying, "Oh my God, that's him!"

I was so surprised to see my son! I'd had a very specific idea of what he would look like, but when he came out he was really his own person. As he was born, we were singing, chanting a wordless Jewish chant, repeating the melody. David was by Gabe's side as the nurses checked him over, then they brought him to me, placed him skin to skin on me, and covered us up.

The midwife made sure Gabe maintained his body temperature, and then he opened his eyes for the first time and looked at me. We were still singing, rubbing him, and holding him.

In the recovery room, my mom and mother-in-law met Gabe while I breast-fed him with the midwife's help. Then my husband and our mothers held him. Soon, we moved to our room—a private room with a balcony—and it was like a party. Australia has such great health care! We were there for five days, with people just hanging out with me and adoring Gabe. I was feeling pretty high, and I recovered quickly from the Cesarean. The midwives thought I had a high pain tolerance, but I just felt so high, and I was determined to get up and care for my son.

I think I'll always have a little grief around the fact that I wasn't at least able to try in this lifetime to push my babies out. But this grief is greatly lightened by the holy, joyful, challenging, and heart-expanding presence of my children in my life. I also felt great knowing that Gabriel's birth helped change hospital policy for the better: When I went back to that hospital two years later to birth my daughter, it had become the norm to let mothers and healthy babies stay together after a Cesarean—because of my experience.

Sometime after Gabe's birth, I told a naturopath classmate that I felt I'd missed out on an essential experience by having a Cesarean section, that I didn't get initiated into motherhood. She told me that *every* birth is a rite of passage. Her insight has been very empowering for me. Having your belly cut open and going through that surgery awake is a huge rite of passage, too. Where I was living, some people had the opinion that if you didn't birth your baby through the birth canal, you weren't as good a mother; you had failed in some way. I had internalized that belief somewhat, and I had to claim my power and experience, like: "Hey, Deborah! Assert your own power. You're just as much a mother as anybody else."

Mama
Maureen Hunt

**Baby**
Madeline
born March 3 at 4:27 p.m.
8 pounds 3 ounces
20¼ inches

# How Birth Was Meant to Be

**With my first baby, I** had an uncomplicated, scheduled Cesarean section at thirty-nine and a half weeks. My baby was breech, and she stayed that way despite the acupressure and moxibustion I'd tried to encourage her to turn.

After the C-section, we were both physically fine, but I felt I had lost my power as a mother. I felt like I didn't give birth to my baby. The doctors pulled her out of me, and the nurses showed her to me briefly, then whisked her away for what felt like an endless hour while they checked her out and sewed me up. After being *one* for so long, then being separated and maneuvered around by doctors and nurses, I felt small and weak emotionally. I felt robbed of a sense of accomplishment. I kept telling myself that the important thing was my health and the health of my baby. I thought I should be satisfied with that. But I wasn't.

Fast-forward six years to the birth of my second child. I was determined to birth my baby myself. I found a clinic that supported vaginal birth after Cesarean (VBAC). I chose the clinic because they had nurse-midwives there, not realizing that I'd have to see an obstetrician for a VBAC. I finally settled on an OB I liked, but the closer my due date came, the more she talked about a C-section.

"Are you sure you are still planning on having a VBAC?" my OB asked, three appointments in a row. "I think your baby is breech right now; maybe we should think about C-section as a possible option," she said, and another time: "You know, you're measuring a little large. Shall we schedule that C-section just in case? Let's see, let me look at my calendar and give you a few dates…"

I needed someone cheering me on, saying, "You can do it!" not someone constantly questioning my decision to pursue a VBAC. At thirty-seven weeks, I switched clinics. Luckily, I live in a big city, and I was able to find a different group of nurse-midwives affiliated with the same hospital.

Immediately, I felt the difference in attitude. The midwives conveyed their belief that birth is natural, and that there are normal variations in the size of both baby and mother, and in the length of labor. They also seemed less concerned that I was thirty-five years and two months old—in the "old woman" category of expectant mothers.

Don't get me wrong: OBs aren't the "bad guys" and nurse-midwives aren't the "good guys." It's just that most healthy pregnant women need the tender-loving, matter-of-fact care of nurse-midwives, while only a minority needs the medical and surgical expertise of an OB.

Having found the supportive midwives I needed, I was ready for a VBAC, I thought. Then, my early labor lasted for seven days, and it was exhausting. For inspiration, my husband and I put up a picture taken the day my first daughter was born.

In that picture, my daughter—who stayed with Grandma while I labored—is one hour old, and her head is resting on my chest. Her head is round and healthy-looking, but not particularly large in the photo, despite the fact that it measured in the 99th percentile at birth and contributed to my needing a C-section. So all I could think about during my early labor was "large head." Subconsciously, I think, I was scared that I couldn't birth this second baby. What if she had a big head, too?

Although I could *say* that I felt confident in my body's ability to give birth naturally, it seemed I hadn't fully let go of my fear that I'd need a C-section again.

Still, I made steady progress in my labor until I got to 5 or 6 centimeters. But there in the final stages, I stalled out for more than seven hours. My husband, Dan, was unbelievable in the support that he gave me. He never left my side, and he gazed into my eyes through each contraction, giving me a focal point.

My midwife took into account that I'm a big-boned, healthy if slightly overweight, athletic 190-pound woman. She knew I drank my raspberry leaf tea, shopped at the natural food co-op, did my prenatal yoga, and sang and danced and was active throughout my pregnancy. The chances of a uterine rupture were minuscule. Knowing that, and seeing on the monitor that my baby was fine, my midwife let me go on laboring a lot longer than an OB would have.

Finally, I decided to get an epidural. With that relief, my hips relaxed immediately and my pelvic bones opened up. I pushed my baby out a few hours later. I did it!! I finally felt like all was right with the world, like this is how birth was meant to be. I had a successful VBAC, and that feels great!

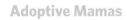
**Adoptive Mamas**
Sarah and Erev Richards

**Baby**
Thea
born April 27 at 8:45 a.m.
8 pounds 13 ounces
21 inches

# The Most Generous Gift

**The phone rang around 3:45** a.m. Surely that meant … Yes! It was the birth parents' cell phone number on caller ID. I answered the phone expectantly. It was Andrew,* calling to tell us that Susie* was in labor. She had been having contractions since late in the evening and they were intensifying. The doula was on her way over, and they would call us when they went to the hospital. I heard a desperate whimper in the background and he told me he had to go. I hung up. My spouse, Erev, and I looked at each other. This was it! Today was the day!

Erev went back to sleep: a smart move. She knew how exhausted we were about to become. I couldn't get back in bed. I went out to install the car seat base in the backseat. I made sure the bag we'd packed for our little girl's brief time in the hospital had everything she'd need, even if we weren't with her. It was so difficult not to be able to be there, knowing she was being born just a ten-minute drive away and we couldn't see her first moments in the world. But we wanted to respect the birth parents' wishes for a private birth. After all, they were giving us their baby.

By 8 a.m. I couldn't stand it anymore. Andrew had said he would call when he and Susie left for the hospital, but that was supposed to be hours ago. Erev busied herself with making the house ready. I called their cell phone. The doula answered and told us Susie was pushing and the baby should be here very soon. I called my parents, my sister,

* The birth parents' names have been changed to respect their privacy.

and a few close friends and told them it was the big day. Then Andrew called. Our baby girl was here!

Around 2 p.m. the birth parents called and asked if we could bring the bag with the formula and clothes to the hospital. We headed for the car, trying to decide whether or not we should meet our little girl before the surrender papers were signed. We decided that even though it would be hard to meet her and then have to go home without her that first night, we couldn't pass up our only opportunity to see her on the day she was born. We arranged for the doula to bring her to a private room on the delivery floor for us to spend some time with her.

The cart rolled in. There was a tiny, swaddled girl with the smoothest skin and most angelic expression of any newborn ever seen. The doula said that she and the nurses agreed they'd never seen a baby born with such smooth skin and "normal" appearance before. She didn't even have a hint of a cone head. We took turns holding her. I instantly fell in love with her nose, deciding it was the cutest part. It was utterly surreal. Erev and I kept looking at each other, not knowing what to say or even how to feel.

That night was hard. We had to go home after our brief visit and somehow *wait* until the next day, when our attorney would come and get all the necessary papers signed. But by late the following morning, everything was taken care of and we got to strap our perfect little girl into her car seat and drive home! Amidst our joy, there was a hint of bittersweetness. We'd all—adoptive parents and birth parents—been in the hospital room together after the papers were signed, and we heard Susie's sobs from the hall after we took the baby from her. Why did someone else have to be so sad so that we could be so happy?

It's been several years since then and we have a happy, healthy little girl, who now has a little brother. We will never forget the day of her birth, and we are grateful each and every day for the beautiful family that was created by the most generous gift on earth.

# Resources

## Pregnancy and Early Parenting Centers

**Belly Bliss**
Denver, Colorado
www.BellyBliss.org
303-399-1191

**Blooma**
Minneapolis/St. Paul, Minnesota
www.Blooma.com
952-848-1111

**Dolphin Yoga and Doula Center**
San Mateo, California
www.DolphinYoga.com
650-888-6996

**Full Bloom**
Athens, Georgia
www.FullBloomParent.com
706-353-3373

Natural Resources
San Francisco, California
www.naturalresources-sf.com
415-550-2611

Prenatal Yoga Center
New York City
www.PrenatalYogaCenter.com
212-362-2985

## Childbirth Education

Birthing from Within
www.birthingfromwithin.com

The Bradley Method of Natural Childbirth
www.bradleybirth.com

Hypnobabies
www.hypnobabies.com

HypnoBirthing: The Mongan Method
www.hypnobirthing.com

Lamaze International
www.lamaze.org

International Childbirth Education Association
ww.icea.org

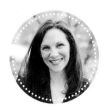

Jennifer Derryberry Mann, freelance writer, editor, and yoga teacher, is passionate about birth, babies, and new (and not-so-new) mamas. Jenni believes in the power of a happy birth story to give families a mindful, healthy beginning. As a writer and editor, she loves covering pregnancy, postnatal care, early parenting, and mindbody care for women and their families. As a certified Forrest Yoga and Yoga Bonding instructor, Jenni helps women navigate the transition to motherhood. She loves teaching expectant mamas, then meeting their babies on the mat in a shared yoga practice, and ultimately helping women create new connections to their core values, core beliefs, and core muscles. Jenni, her husband, Scotty, and their two daughters, Anabel and Alia, make their home in Athens, Georgia. Visit JenniferDerryberry.com for more birth stories and mama mindbody care.